NUTRITIONAL FOOD

DURING PREGNANCY

INTRODUCTION

A woman's body goes through major changes during pregnancy to support the growth and development of a new life, making it a special moment for her body.. During this period, proper nutrition is crucial for both the mother and the developing foetus. Preventing issues like gestational diabetes, preeclampsia, and preterm birth during pregnancy can be accomplished by eating a healthy, balanced diet.

Consuming nutrients, vitamins, and minerals that are needed for the foetus's healthy growth and development throughout pregnancy is referred to as nutritional diet.A healthy and balanced diet during pregnancy should contain a variety of foods from all the major food groups, such as fruits, vegetables, whole grains, lean protein, and low-fat dairy products. Additionally, it's crucial to stay hydrated by drinking lots of water all day long.

The essential nutrients folic acid, iron, calcium, and omega-3 fatty acids are some of the ones that are most important during pregnancy. Folic acid helps to avoid brain and spinal birth defects, whereas iron is necessary for the creation of red blood cells and the supply of oxygen to the foetus. The development of the baby's bones and teeth depends on calcium, while the growth of the baby's brain and eyes depends on omega-3 fatty acids.

Some foods, such as raw or undercooked meat, fish, or eggs, unpasteurized dairy products, and some fish types with high mercury levels should be avoided by expectant mothers.

Overall, a healthy and balanced diet is essential for both the mother and the growing foetus during pregnancy. By consuming nutrient-rich foods and avoiding harmful substances, pregnant women can help ensure a healthy pregnancy and the optimal growth and development of their baby.

Eating a healthy, balanced diet is important for everyone, but it's especially crucial for pregnant women. The food you eat during pregnancy not only fuels your body but also provides the essential nutrients your growing baby needs to develop properly.

However, not all foods are created equal, and consuming processed or unhealthy foods can have negative consequences for both you and your baby. That's where real food comes in. Real food is anything that is entire, unprocessed, and as close to its original state as possible. These foods are packed with nutrients and offer a range of health benefits.

This section will discuss the value of real food during pregnancy and offer helpful advice and guidance to help you increase the amount of genuine food in your diet. We'll go through everything you need to know to eat healthily and nurture yourself and your developing baby during this exciting time, from necessary nutrients to genuine food

alternatives.

IMPORTANCE OF NUTRITIONAL FOOD DURING PREGNANCY

A healthy diet is crucial during pregnancy for both the mother and the developing foetus. Here are some reasons why:

1. **Supports Healthy Foetal Development:** The food you eat provides your growing baby with the necessary nutrients for healthy development. Adequate intake of nutrients such as protein, calcium, iron, and folate can help prevent birth defects, low birth weight, and other complications. The following essential nutrients are crucial for fetal growth:

   - **Protein**: The growth of fetal tissues and organs, including the brain, heart, and lungs, depends on protein. It also supports the development and repair of maternal tissues. Meat, poultry, fish, eggs, dairy products, legumes, and nuts are all excellent sources of protein.

- [ ] **Calcium:** The development of healthy teeth and strong bones in the foetus depends on calcium. Additionally, it aids in nerve and muscle function. Almonds, tofu, leafy green vegetables, dairy products, and dairy products are all great sources of calcium.

- [ ] **Iron:** Red blood cells, which deliver oxygen to the foetus, are produced only when iron is present in the body. Anaemia, premature labour, and low birth weight can all result from iron deficiency during pregnancy. Excellent sources of iron include red meat, poultry, fish, leafy green vegetables, and fortified cereals.

- [ ] **Folate:** Folate is essential for the development of the foetal neural tube and can help avoid birth abnormalities. Red blood cell production is influenced by it as well. Leafy green vegetables, citrus fruits, legumes, and fortified cereals are all excellent sources of folate.

☐ **Omega-3 Fatty Acids**: Omega-3 fatty acids, particularly DHA, are important for foetal brain and eye development. Omega-3 fatty acids are abundant in fatty fish like salmon, sardines, and tuna as well as walnuts and flaxseed.

The best method to guarantee adequate consumption of these crucial nutrients is to eat a balanced diet that consists of a variety of whole, unprocessed foods. In some cases, prenatal supplements may be recommended to ensure adequate intake of certain nutrients. It's best to speak with a healthcare professional before taking any supplements, though.

2. **Boosts Maternal Health:** Proper nutrition during pregnancy can also benefit the mother's health. A healthy diet can lower your chances of developing pregnancy-related conditions such as gestational diabetes and pre-eclampsia.

Here are some ways that a balanced diet can help boost maternal health:

- ☐ Reduces the Risk of Pregnancy-Related Complications: Pregnancy-related illnesses such as gestational diabetes, pre-eclampsia, and high blood pressure can be lessened by eating a healthy, balanced diet.Both the mother and the child may suffer harmful effects as a result of these difficulties.

- [ ] Supports Healthy Weight Gain: Gaining weight during pregnancy is normal and necessary, but excessive weight gain can increase the risk of pregnancy-related complications. Eating a nutritious diet can help support healthy weight gain and prevent excessive weight gain.

- [ ] Provides Energy and Vitality: Pregnancy can be exhausting, and proper nutrition can help provide energy and vitality to get through the day. Consuming a well-balanced diet full of a range of nutritious foods can help regulate blood sugar levels and provide you constant energy all day.

- [ ] Improves Gut Health: Pregnancy can sometimes lead to digestive issues such as constipation and bloating. Consuming a diet high in fiber-rich foods, such as fruits, vegetables, and whole grains, can help maintain digestive health and promote gut health.

☐ Supports Mental Health: Proper nutrition can also support mental health during pregnancy. Pregnancy-related depression and anxiety may be decreased by eating a balanced diet that contains foods high in omega-3 fatty acids, like fatty fish and walnuts.

In summary, a healthy, balanced diet during pregnancy can help boost maternal health by reducing the risk of pregnancy-related complications, supporting healthy weight gain, providing energy and vitality, improving gut health, and supporting mental health.

3. **Helps with Postpartum Recovery:** A healthy diet during pregnancy helps with postpartum recovery. Adequate intake of nutrients such as iron and protein can help with postpartum healing and breastfeeding.

   Proper nutrition during pregnancy can also benefit postpartum recovery. After giving birth, the body undergoes significant physical and hormonal changes, and a healthy diet can help support the healing process. Here are some ways that proper nutrition can help with postpartum recovery:

   - ☐ Supports Breastfeeding: Breastfeeding is an excellent source of nutrition for babies, and a healthy diet can help support milk production and ensure that the baby receives all the nutrients they need. It's important for breastfeeding mothers to consume enough calories and stay hydrated to support milk production.

☐ Provides Energy for Recovery: The postpartum period can be physically demanding, and a healthy diet can provide the energy and nutrients needed for the body to heal and recover. Eating a balanced diet that includes plenty of whole foods can help support energy levels and provide the necessary nutrients for recovery.

☐ Supports Hormonal Balance: Hormonal fluctuations are common after giving birth, and proper nutrition can help support hormonal balance. A diet rich in healthy fats, such as those found in avocados and nuts, helps boost the production and balance of hormones.

- ☐ Promotes Healing: Zinc and vitamin C are two minerals that are crucial for wound healing. The body may acquire the nutrients it needs to mend and recover by consuming a diet rich in fruits, vegetables, lean protein, and whole grains.

- ☐ Prevents Postpartum Depression: After giving birth, postpartum depression is a common disorder that can develop. Postpartum depression may be avoided with a balanced diet that includes foods high in omega-3 fatty acids, like fatty fish and flaxseed.

4. **Improves Mood and Energy Levels:** Proper nutrition can also improve mood and energy levels during pregnancy. Consuming a diet high in whole foods can support blood sugar stabilisation and offer enduring energy throughout the day.

Proper nutrition during pregnancy helps to improve mood and energy levels. Hormonal changes, physical stress, and the demands of pregnancy can often leave expecting mothers feeling tired and moody. A healthy diet can provide the necessary nutrients to help maintain a stable mood and energy levels throughout pregnancy. Here are some ways that a balanced diet can help improve mood and energy levels:

☐ Stabilises Blood Sugar Levels: Eating regular meals that include a balance of protein, healthy fats, and complex carbohydrates can help stabilise blood sugar levels. This can help prevent energy crashes and mood swings that can occur when blood sugar levels are unstable.

☐ Provides B Vitamins: B vitamins are crucial for regulating mood and supplying energy.

Foods that are rich in B vitamins include whole grains, leafy green vegetables, and lean protein.

- [ ] Provides Iron: The creation of haemoglobin, which transports oxygen throughout the body, depends on iron. Fatigue and poor energy levels can be caused by an iron shortage. Lean red meat, spinach, and lentils are a few examples of foods that are high in iron.

- [ ] Provides Omega-3 Fatty Acids: It has been demonstrated that omega-3 fatty acids enhance mood and lower the risk of depression. Foods high in omega-3s include flaxseed, walnuts, and fatty fish.

- [ ] Provides Antioxidants: Vitamins C and E and other antioxidants can aid in preventing oxidative stress from damaging cells. Berries, citrus fruits, and dark leafy greens are examples of foods high in antioxidants.

In summary, a balanced diet that includes a variety of whole foods can help improve mood and energy levels during pregnancy. Eating regular meals that include protein, healthy fats, and complex carbohydrates can help stabilise blood sugar levels and prevent energy crashes. Foods that are rich in B vitamins, iron, omega-3 fatty acids, and antioxidants can help support energy levels and improve mood.

5. **Sets Healthy Eating Habits for the Future:** Eating a healthy diet during pregnancy can also set the foundation for healthy eating habits in the future. A balanced diet can help establish healthy habits for both the mother and the child.

Eating a healthy diet during pregnancy not only benefits the mother and baby during pregnancy but can also set the stage for healthy eating habits in the future. Developing healthy eating habits during pregnancy can help ensure that the mother and child continue to make healthy food choices in the future. Here are some ways that a healthy diet during pregnancy can set healthy eating habits for the future:

1. Establishes a Healthy Relationship with Food: A balanced diet can promote a positive relationship with food when consumed throughout pregnancy. Eating whole foods that are nutrient-dense and satisfying can help the mother and baby feel their best and develop a positive relationship with food.

2. Models Healthy Eating Habits: Children learn by example, and seeing their mother make healthy food choices can help establish healthy eating habits for life. By modelling healthy eating habits during pregnancy, the mother can set a positive example for her child.

3. Introduces a Variety of Foods: Pregnant women can offer a range of foods to their unborn children through a balanced diet. Introducing a variety of foods can help establish a diverse palate and encourage the child to try new foods in the future.

4. Encourages Family Meals: Eating together as a family can help establish healthy eating habits for life. By prioritising family meals during pregnancy, the mother can establish

a routine of eating together as a family and promote healthy eating habits.

5. Prioritises Nutrient-Dense Foods: A healthy diet during pregnancy prioritises nutrient-dense foods that provide the necessary nutrients for the mother and baby. Prioritising nutrient-dense foods can help establish a pattern of making healthy food choices and prioritising whole foods.

A healthy diet is crucial during pregnancy for both the mother and the developing foetus. It can support healthy foetal development, boost maternal health, aid in postpartum recovery, improve mood and energy levels, and set healthy eating habits for the future.

ESSENTIAL NUTRIENTS FOR PREGNANCY

A woman's body needs more nutrients during pregnancy to support the growth and development of the fetus. To make sure that the mother and unborn child receive all the nutrients they require throughout pregnancy, it is crucial to eat a balanced and healthy diet. Here are some essential nutrients for pregnancy:

1. **Folic Acid:**The neural tube, which eventually develops into the baby's brain and spinal cord, requires the B vitamin folic acid to function properly. When the neural tube is developing during the first trimester of pregnancy, adequate folic acid consumption is particularly crucial. Spina bifida is one example of a neural tube abnormality that can occur if the neural tube does not develop properly..

For pregnant women, 600–800 mcg of folic acid per day is advised. To ensure adequate levels of the nutrient in their bodies, women who intend to become pregnant should begin taking folic acid supplements at least one month prior to conception.

Leafy green vegetables like spinach and kale, citrus fruits, beans, peas, and fortified cereals are among foods that are high in folic acid. However, it can be difficult to obtain the recommended amount of folic acid from food alone, which is why folic acid supplements are often recommended.

Folic acid provides additional advantages for both the mother and the unborn child in addition to lowering the chance of neural tube abnormalities. As a result of the increased blood volume during pregnancy, it can aid in preventing anaemia, which is a common problem. The creation of DNA and RNA, which are necessary for the growth and development of the baby's cells, is another function of folic acid.

It is important to note that not all women can absorb folic acid as easily as others, so some may require higher doses of the nutrient. Women who suffer from certain illnesses, such as celiac disease or inflammatory bowel disease, may have trouble absorbing folic acid and may need additional supplements.

Overall, folic acid is an essential nutrient for pregnant women to ensure the healthy development of their baby. Women who are planning to become pregnant should speak with their healthcare provider about the appropriate dosage and timing of folic acid supplementation.

2. **Iron**:Because it contributes to the production of haemoglobin, a protein found in red blood cells that delivers oxygen to the foetus, iron is a crucial nutrient during pregnancy. A woman's blood volume rises by roughly 50% during pregnancy, necessitating a higher iron intake to sustain the extra red blood cells.For pregnant women, a daily intake of 27 milligrams of iron is advised. However, many women do not consume enough iron through their diet alone, and may require supplementation to prevent iron deficiency anaemia.

Good dietary sources of iron include red meat, poultry, fish, beans, lentils, spinach, and fortified cereals. Vitamin C can also enhance the absorption of iron from plant-based foods, so consuming foods rich in vitamin C, such as citrus fruits and tomatoes, along with iron-rich foods can help to increase iron absorption.

Preterm birth, low birth weight, and developmental delays in the foetus are just a few issues that can arise from iron deficiency anaemia during pregnancy.. Anaemia due to iron deficiency is characterised by weakness, weariness, and pale skin.

Women who are at a higher risk of iron deficiency anaemia during pregnancy include those who have a history of anaemia, are carrying twins or multiples, have a history of heavy menstrual bleeding, or have a vegan or vegetarian diet. These women may require additional iron supplementation or monitoring to ensure that they are getting enough iron.

It is important to note that taking too much iron can be harmful, so women should not take iron supplements without consulting with their healthcare provider first. Iron supplements can also cause constipation and nausea, so it is important to take them with food and drink plenty of water.

In conclusion, iron is an essential nutrient during pregnancy to support the production of red blood cells and prevent iron deficiency anaemia. Women should try to eat a balanced diet that contains foods high in iron and, if necessary, talk to their healthcare professional about the right amount and timing of iron supplementation.

3. **Calcium**:Due to its critical function in the growth of the baby's bones, teeth, muscles, and nervous system, calcium is a crucial nutrient throughout pregnancy. The mother's food provides calcium throughout pregnancy, which the growing baby needs to create strong bones and teeth.

Depending on characteristics including age and other considerations, pregnant women should consume 1000–1300 mg of calcium every day. Dairy products, such as milk, cheese, and yoghourt, leafy green vegetables, such as kale and collard greens, as well as fortified cereals and juices are all excellent sources of calcium.

Women who do not consume enough calcium through their diet may require supplementation to meet their needs. However, it's crucial to adhere to the daily calcium recommendations because consuming too much calcium can cause constipation, kidney stones, and other problems.

In addition to supporting the baby's development, calcium also plays a role in maintaining the mother's bone density. During pregnancy, the baby's growing bones absorb calcium from the mother's bones, which can lead to a loss of bone density. Adequate calcium intake can help to prevent this and reduce the risk of osteoporosis later in life.

It is significant to note that vitamin D improves calcium absorption, which is why many prenatal supplements include both calcium and vitamin D. Fatty seafood, such as salmon and tuna, and fortified foods, such milk and cereal, are good dietary sources of vitamin D.

Women who are at a higher risk of calcium deficiency during pregnancy include those who have a vegan or vegetarian diet, have lactose intolerance or milk allergy, or have a history of bone loss or fractures. These women may require additional supplementation or monitoring to ensure that they are getting enough calcium.

In conclusion, calcium is an essential nutrient during pregnancy to support the baby's development and maintain the mother's bone density. Women should aim to consume a balanced diet that includes calcium-rich foods and speak with their healthcare provider about the appropriate dosage and timing of calcium supplementation if needed.

4. **Protein:**Protein is an essential nutrient during pregnancy, as it is needed for the growth and development of the baby's cells, tissues, and organs. Protein is also important for the growth and maintenance of the mother's own tissues, such as the uterus and breast tissue.

Protein for pregnant women should be consumed in amounts of 71 grams daily, which is a little bit more than for non-pregnant women. Lean meats, poultry, fish, beans, lentils, eggs, and dairy products are all excellent sources of protein.

To make sure that the body is receiving all of the essential amino acids required for growth and development, it is crucial to consume a range of protein sources. All of the essential amino acids are present in animal-based proteins like meat, poultry, and dairy products, however plant-based proteins like beans and lentils may require the addition of other protein sources to provide all of the essential amino acids.

Some women may require additional protein during pregnancy, such as those who are carrying twins or multiples or those who are underweight or have a history of low birth weight babies. In these cases, a healthcare provider may recommend a higher protein intake or supplementation to ensure that the body is getting enough protein to support the baby's growth and development.

It is crucial to remember that consuming too much protein during pregnancy can also be hazardous because it can cause dehydration, constipation, and other issues. Therefore, it is important to speak with a healthcare provider about the appropriate amount of protein for individual needs.

During pregnancy, protein is a crucial component for the mother's tissues as well as the baby's growth and development. In addition to talking to their healthcare physician about the right quantity of protein for their specific needs, women should try to eat a balanced diet that includes a variety of protein sources.

5. **Vitamin D**:Due to its critical function in the growth and development of the baby's bones and teeth as well as its support of the immune system, vitamin D is an essential supplement for expectant mothers. It

also facilitates the body's absorption of calcium, which is necessary for healthy bones.

The daily recommended allowance of vitamin D during pregnancy is between 600 and 800 international units (IU). Fatty fish, such as salmon and tuna, egg yolks, fortified dairy products, and supplements are all excellent sources of vitamin D.

Nevertheless, many people do not get enough vitamin D through diet alone, particularly if they live in places with little sunlight or have darker skin, which might hinder the body's capacity to generate vitamin D from sunlight. Therefore, it is recommended that pregnant women take a daily vitamin D supplement to ensure adequate intake. Vitamin D deficiency during pregnancy has been linked to a higher risk of complications, including gestational diabetes, preeclampsia, and preterm birth. It has also been associated with a higher risk of the baby developing rickets, a condition that causes weak and brittle bones.

In addition to a healthy diet and vitamin D supplementation, pregnant women can also increase their vitamin D levels by spending time in the sun, typically between 10-30 minutes per day, with exposed skin and without sunscreen, depending on the individual's skin type and location. However, it is important to avoid getting sunburned or overheated.

Vitamin D is an important nutrient for pregnant women to support the growth and development of the baby's bones, teeth, and immune system. Women should aim to consume a balanced diet rich in vitamin D, take a daily vitamin D supplement, and speak with their healthcare provider about the appropriate amount of vitamin D for their individual needs. Additionally, spending time in the sun can also help boost vitamin D levels, but should be done safely and without risking sun damage.

6. **Omega-3 fatty acids** are a type of essential fatty acid that are important for overall health, including during pregnancy. Since the body is unable to generate them on its own, they are regarded as "essential" and must be received through diet or supplements

Alpha-linolenic acid (ALA), eicosapentaenoic acid (EPA), and docosahexaenoic acid (DHA) are the three different kinds of omega-3 fatty acids. While ALA is found in plant-based sources like flaxseeds and chia seeds, EPA and DHA are found in fatty seafood like salmon and tuna.

Omega-3 fatty acids are essential for the baby's brain and eyes to grow throughout pregnancy. They also support the immune system, reduce inflammation, and may help to reduce the risk of preterm birth.

The recommended daily intake of omega-3 fatty acids during pregnancy is at least 200-300 milligrams (mg) of DHA, which can be obtained through a combination of dietary sources and supplements. However, pregnant women should be cautious about consuming high levels of certain types of fish that may contain high levels of mercury, which can be harmful to the developing baby's nervous system.

In addition to consuming fatty fish, pregnant women can also obtain omega-3 fatty acids through supplements, such as fish oil or algae-based supplements. It is important to speak with a healthcare provider before taking any supplements, as they can interact with certain mecications or have side effects.

Omega-3 fatty acids are an important nutrient for pregnant women to support the development of the baby's brain and eyes, as well as overall health. In addition to consuming an adequate amount of omega-3 supplements for their particular needs, women should strive to eat a balanced diet rich in these fats from both animal and plant sources. They should also discuss this with their healthcare professional.

7. **Vitamin C:**Vitamin The vitamin C is a necessary nutrient that is important for sustaining general health, especially during pregnancy. This water-soluble vitamin is essential for collagen synthesis, immune function, wound healing, and

iron absorption, among other things. During pregnancy, the recommended daily intake of vitamin C is slightly higher than for non-pregnant women.

Here are some of the reasons why vitamin C is important during pregnancy:

☐ Immune System Support

Vitamin C is well-known for its immune-boosting properties, and this is especially important during pregnancy when a woman's immune system is already under stress. Vitamin C helps protect against infections and illnesses that can harm both the mother and the growing foetus.

☐ Collagen Synthesis

Collagen is a protein that helps build and maintain healthy tissues in the body, including those in the skin, bones, and blood vessels. Vitamin C is essential for collagen synthesis, and during pregnancy, it is particularly important for foetal bone and cartilage development.

☐ Iron Absorption

Iron is another essential nutrient during pregnancy, as it is required for the formation of red blood cells. As significant sources of iron for pregnant women as spinach and lentils, vitamin C improves the absorption of iron from plant-based sources.

☐ Antioxidant Properties

Strong antioxidants like vitamin C help to ward off harm from dangerous chemicals known as free radicals. During pregnancy, the body is under increased oxidative stress, and vitamin C can help reduce the risk of oxidative damage to the developing foetus.

☐ Wound Healing

During pregnancy, the body undergoes a lot of changes, and wound healing is an essential process that helps repair and regenerate tissues. Vitamin C is essential for wound healing, and it helps support healthy skin and tissue repair.

In conclusion, vitamin C is a critical nutrient during pregnancy, and it is important for maintaining overall health and supporting the healthy development of the foetus. Women who are expecting should make an effort to eat a balanced diet with lots of fruits and vegetables, which are great providers of vitamin C. If necessary, a prenatal vitamin supplement can also provide additional vitamin C to support a healthy pregnancy.

NUTRITIONAL FOOD SOURCES

Eating a balanced and nutritious diet is essential for overall health and well-being. Essential nutrients such as vitamins, minerals, and antioxidants play vital roles in many bodily functions, from maintaining a healthy immune system to supporting healthy bone growth. Here are some real food sources of essential nutrients that can help you meet your daily requirements:

1. **Meat, poultry and fish:Meat,**Fish anc poultry are great providers of B vitamins, iron, zinc, and high-quality protein, among other nutrients. These foods provide a range of essential nutrients that are important for maintaining overall health and well-being.

Here are some of the key nutrients found in meat, poultry, and fish:

☐ Protein

Meat, poultry, and fish are excellent sources of high-quality protein, which is essential for building and repairing tissues in the body. In addition, protein is essential for the body's production of enzymes, hormones, and other critical compounds.

☐ Iron

For the body to transfer oxygen and maintain healthy blood cells, iron is a necessary mineral. Red meat is one of the meals with the highest iron content, and fish, poultry, and meat are some of the finest dietary sources of iron.

☐ Zinc

Zinc is a necessary mineral that aids in DNA synthesis, wound healing, and immunological function. Meat, poultry, and fish are excellent sources of zinc, with oysters being one of the richest sources of this mineral.

☐ B Vitamins

B vitamins, such as vitamin B12, which is necessary for healthy neurological function and the production of red blood cells, are abundant in meat, poultry, and fish. Other B vitamins found in these foods include thiamin, riboflavin, niacin, and vitamin B6, which are important for energy production and metabolism.

☐ Omega-3 Fatty Acids

Omega-3 fatty acids, which are crucial for heart health, cognitive function, and lowering inflammation in the body, are found in abundance in some fish varieties, including salmon, mackerel, and tuna. Additionally essential for foetal growth during pregnancy, these fatty acids.

While meat, poultry, and fish are good providers of nutrients, it's crucial to choose lean cuts of meat and limit the consumption of red and processed meats in order to lower the chance of developing chronic diseases like cancer and heart disease. Choosing fish that are low in mercury and other contaminants is also important for overall health.

The bottom line is that meat, poultry, and fish are great suppliers of a variety of vital nutrients, including as protein, iron, zinc, B vitamins, and omega-3 fatty acids. Incorporating these foods into a balanced and varied diet can help ensure that you are getting the nutrients you need to maintain optimal health and well-being.

2. **Dairy products**:Protein, calcium, vitamin D, and other vital elements can all be found in large quantities in dairy products. These nutrients are important for maintaining strong bones, healthy teeth, and supporting overall health and well-being. Here are some of the key nutrients found in dairy products:

☐ Calcium

A crucial component for the development and maintenance of healthy bones and teeth is calcium.

Dairy products such as milk, yoghourt, and cheese are some of the best dietary sources of calcium, with one cup of milk providing approximately 30% of the daily recommended intake for adults.

☐ Vitamin D

Vitamin D is crucial for maintaining strong bones, teeth, and muscles. It also supports immune system health. While getting vitamin D from the sun is one way to get it, fortified dairy products like milk and yoghurt also contain it.

☐ Protein

The body needs high-quality protein for tissue growth and repair, and dairy products are a superb supply of this protein. In addition, protein is essential for the body's production of enzymes, hormones, and other critical compounds.

☐ Other Nutrients

Dairy products contain other essential nutrients, such as vitamin B12, which is crucial for proper neurological function and the generation of red blood cells, and riboflavin, which is crucial for energy production and metabolism, in addition to calcium, vitamin D, and protein.

It is crucial to note that while dairy products can provide important nutrients, they can also be high in saturated fat and calories. Choosing low-fat or fat-free dairy products and limiting intake to recommended servings can help ensure that you are getting the health benefits of dairy while also maintaining a healthy diet.

3. **Eggs:**Eggs are a highly nutritious and versatile food that is widely consumed all over the world. They are a great source of protein, healthy fats, vitamins, and minerals. In fact, they are considered one of the most nutritious foods available. Here's a

closer look at the nutrients found in eggs and their benefits.

☐ Protein:

One big egg has about 6 grams of protein, making it a fantastic source of protein. All nine of the essential amino acids are present in good quality in the protein found in eggs. Our bodies require amino acids, which are the building blocks of protein, in order to assemble and repair tissues. Protein is also essential for maintaining muscle mass and keeping our bodies functioning properly.

☐ Healthy Fats:

Additionally, monounsaturated and polyunsaturated fats, which are found in eggs, are rich sources of healthful fats. As they can help lower cholesterol levels, reduce inflammation, and promote brain function, these fats are crucial for maintaining excellent health.

☐ Vitamins:

Several vitamins, such as vitamin A, vitamin D, and vitamin B12, are abundant in eggs. The health of your eyes depends on vitamin A, and your bones and immune system depend on vitamin D. Red blood cells and healthy nerve cells both depend on vitamin B12.

☐ Minerals:

Minerals including selenium, phosphorus, and iron are also abundant in eggs. While phosphorus is critical for keeping strong bones and teeth, iron is crucial for carrying oxygen throughout the body. Selenium is important for thyroid function and helps protect against oxidative stress.

Eggs are an excellent source of nutrition, providing protein, healthy fats, vitamins, and minerals. They are a versatile food that can be enjoyed in many different ways, making them a great addition to any diet. If you're looking for a nutritious and convenient food, eggs are definitely worth considering.

4. **Legumes:**Legumes are a family of plants that includes beans, peas, lentils, and chickpeas. They are a nutritious and affordable source of protein, fibre, vitamins, and minerals. Here's a closer look at the nutrients found in legumes and their benefits.

☐ Protein:

An great source of plant-based protein is legumes. One cup of cooked beans contains approximately 15 grams of protein, making them a great alternative to meat for vegetarians and vegans. Legume protein is also considered "incomplete" because it lacks some of the essential amino acids. However, by combining legumes with grains, such as rice or bread, you can create a complete protein source.

☐ Fibre:

Legumes are an excellent source of dietary fibre, including both soluble and insoluble fibres. Insoluble fibre helps support good digestion and help prevent constipation, while soluble fibre can help lower cholesterol and control blood sugar.

☐ Vitamins:

Legumes are a rich source of several vitamins, including folate, thiamine, and vitamin B6. Folate is crucial for cell development and growth, and pregnant women should consume plenty of it to avoid birth abnormalities. Thiamine is essential for energy production, while vitamin B6 is important for brain development and immune function.

☐ Minerals:

Iron, magnesium, and potassium are all minerals that are abundant in legumes.. Iron is important for transporting oxygen throughout the body, while magnesium is essential for bone health and muscle function. Potassium plays a crucial role in controlling blood pressure and preserving fluid balance.

In addition to their nutritional benefits, legumes are also an affordable and versatile food that can be incorporated into many different dishes. They are a staple food in many cultures around the world and can be cooked in a variety of ways, including boiled, roasted, or mashed. Legumes can also be used to make vegetarian burgers, soups, and stews.

Legumes are a nutrient-dense food that provides protein, fibre, vitamins, and minerals. They are an excellent choice for vegetarians and vegans, and they can also be enjoyed by anyone looking to add more plant-based foods to their diet. With their versatility and affordability, legumes are a great choice for anyone looking to improve their health through diet.

5. **Whole grain:**Nuts and seeds are a great source of nutrients that offer a variety of health benefits. They are rich in healthy fats, protein, fibre, vitamins, and minerals, all of which are important for maintaining good health.

The high concentration of beneficial fats, such as monounsaturated and polyunsaturated fats, found in nuts and seeds is one of its main advantages. These fats can help to reduce inflammation in the body, lower cholesterol levels, and improve heart health. Some of the best sources of healthy fats are almonds, walnuts, pistachios, flaxseeds, chia seeds, and hemp seeds.

Nuts and seeds are a great choice for vegetarians and vegans because they are a fantastic source of plant-based protein. They can help you feel full and satisfied since they include all the essential amino acids your body needs to build and repair tissues. Some of the best sources of protein in nuts and seeds include almonds, pumpkin seeds, hemp seeds, and peanuts.

In addition to healthy fats and protein, nuts and seeds are also rich in fibre, vitamins, and minerals. Fibre helps to keep the digestive system running smoothly and can lower the risk of chronic diseases such as heart disease, diabetes, and certain types of cancer. Vitamins and minerals found in nuts and seeds include vitamin E, magnesium, phosphorus, and potassium, all of which play important roles in maintaining good health.

One of the great things about nuts and seeds is that they are easy to incorporate into your diet. You can snack on a handful of almonds or pumpkin seeds, add flaxseeds or chia seeds to your smoothies or yoghurt, or sprinkle some sunflower seeds on your salad. You can also use nut butters such as almond butter or peanut butter as a healthy spread on toast or crackers.

Nuts and seeds are a nutritious and delicious addition to any diet. By incorporating a variety of nuts and seeds into your meals and snacks, you can enjoy their many health benefits and support your overall health and well-being.

6. **Fruits and vegetables:** are an essential source of nutrients that offer a wide range of health benefits. They are abundant in antioxidants, fiber, vitamins,

and minerals, all of which are crucial for sustaining excellent health.

One of the most notable benefits of fruits and vegetables is their high content of vitamins and minerals. These nutrients are crucial for many biological processes, including maintaining healthy bones, boosting the immune system, and warding off chronic illnesses like cancer and heart disease. Some of the best sources of vitamins and minerals in fruits and vegetables include leafy greens like spinach and kale, berries like blueberries and strawberries, and citrus fruits like oranges and grapefruits.

In addition to vitamins and minerals, fruits and vegetables are also a great source of fibre. Fibre can decrease cholesterol and aid to maintain healthy blood sugar levels in addition to supporting a healthy digestive system. Some of the best sources of fibre in fruits and vegetables include apples, bananas, broccoli, and sweet potatoes.

Another important benefit of fruits and vegetables is their high content of antioxidants. Against oxidative stress, which can result in chronic diseases like cancer and heart disease, antioxidants aid in defending the body. Some of the best sources of antioxidants in fruits and vegetables include blueberries, raspberries, blackberries, and dark leafy greens like kale and spinach.

Finally, fruits and vegetables are versatile and easy to incorporate into your diet. You can enjoy them raw or cooked, in salads, smoothies, soups, stir-fries, and more. You can also use them as a healthy snack throughout the day, or as a nutritious addition to any meal.

In conclusion, fruits and vegetables are an essential source of nutrients that offer a wide range of health benefits. You may improve your general health and wellbeing, lower your chance of developing chronic diseases, and boost your diet by including a range of fruits and vegetables.

THE ROLE OF SUPPLEMENTS DURING PREGNANCY

Supplements can play a significant role in meeting nutrient needs, especially for individuals who have dietary restrictions, certain health conditions, or are unable to consume enough nutrients from their diet alone. It's crucial to remember that supplements shouldn't be used in place of a healthy, balanced diet and should only be used as directed by a healthcare provider.

Here are some key points to consider about the role of supplements in meeting nutrient needs:

1. Supplements can provide essential vitamins and minerals that may be lacking in the diet: Despite our best efforts to eat a varied and balanced diet, it can be challenging to consume enough of certain nutrients. For example, people who follow a vegan or vegetarian diet may have difficulty getting

enough vitamin B12, which is mostly found in animal-based foods. In this case, taking a B12 supplement can help meet the daily recommended intake.

2. Supplements can help address nutrient deficiencies: If blood tests indicate that someone has a deficiency in a certain nutrient, such as iron or vitamin D, supplements may be recommended to help bring levels back to normal. To decide on the proper dosage and duration of supplementation, it's crucial to see a healthcare specialist.

3. Supplements may be beneficial for certain health conditions: Some health conditions, such as osteoporosis or arthritis, may benefit from supplements such as calcium or omega-3 fatty acids. Again, choosing the right type and dosage of supplements requires consultation with a healthcare provider.

4. Supplements should not be used in place of a healthy diet: While supplements can be helpful in meeting nutrient needs, they should not be viewed as a substitute for a healthy, balanced diet. Whole foods contain a wide range of nutrients and other beneficial compounds that cannot be replicated in supplement form. To make sure that you're getting enough nutrients, you should concentrate on eating a range of entire meals.

5. Not all supplements are created equal: The quality and safety of supplements can vary widely. It's important to choose supplements from reputable companies that have undergone third-party testing to ensure quality and purity. Additionally, certain supplements may interact with medications or have negative side effects, so it's important to discuss any supplement use with a healthcare professional.

In conclusion, supplements can play an important role in meeting nutrient needs, but they should be used judiciously and under the guidance of a healthcare professional. A healthy, balanced diet should always be the foundation of good nutrition.

SAMPLE MEAL PLAN FOR PREGNANT

A nutritious, well-balanced diet is essential during pregnancy because it helps the mother maintain her own health while also giving the baby the nutrition it needs to grow. A well-planned meal plan can ensure that pregnant women get all the nutrients they need, including protein, iron, folate, calcium, and omega-3 fatty acids. Here is a sample meal plan for pregnancy:

1. **Breakfast:Breakfast:**Breakfast is an essential meal for pregnant women as it helps provide the necessary nutrients and energy for both the mother and the developing foetus. Pre-eclampsia, gestational diabetes, and low birth weight are just a few of the pregnancy issues that can be lowered with a healthy breakfast. We will go through some

easy meal plans for a nutritious breakfast in this part.

Why is Breakfast Important during Pregnancy?

The mother's body needs more nutrients during pregnancy to support the development and growth of the foetus. Breakfast is an important meal as it helps provide the necessary energy and nutrients to support the mother's health and the growth of the foetus. Lack of blood sugar can result from skipping breakfast and induce weariness, wooziness, and nausea.

Simple Breakfast Meal Plan Ideas for Pregnancy

- ☐ Banana with peanut butter on whole-wheat toast.

Complex carbohydrates are provided by whole-grain toast, while protein and good fats are present in peanut butter. In addition to adding a natural sweetness, bananas contain vital nutrients including potassium and folate. Simply toast a slice of whole-grain bread, spread peanut butter on top, and add sliced banana for a nutritious and satisfying breakfast.

☐ Greek Yoghourt with Berries and Almonds

Greek yoghurt is a great source of protein and calcium, while berries are high in antioxidants and fibre. Almonds add a crunchy texture and provide healthy fats and carbohydrates. Simply mix together a cup of Greek yoghurt with a handful of berries and a serving of almonds for a quick and healthy breakfast.

☐ Scrambled Eggs with Spinach and Whole Grain Toast

Eggs are a good source of protein and key nutrients including choline, which is crucial for the growth of the foetus's brain. Spinach is a great source of iron and folic acid, which are important for foetal growth and development. Whole-grain toast provides complex carbohydrates. Simply scramble two eggs with a handful of spinach and serve with a slice of whole-grain toast for a filling and nutritious breakfast.

☐ Smoothie with Greek Yogurt and Berries

Adding a variety of fruits and veggies to your morning meal is easy with smoothies. Greek yoghurt provides protein and calcium, while berries are high in antioxidants and fibre. Simply blend together a cup of Greek yoghurt, a handful of berries, and a liquid of your choice (such as almond milk or coconut water) for a nutritious and refreshing breakfast.

In conclusion, a healthy breakfast is important during pregnancy as it provides the necessary nutrients and energy for both the mother and the developing foetus. Pregnant women can make sure they are getting the nutrients they need to stay

healthy and support the growth and development of

their baby by implementing easy meal planning into

their morning routine.

2. **Snacks:** It's crucial to make sure you're getting all the nutrients you need during pregnancy to support the healthy growth of your unborn child.Snacks can be a great way to supplement your meals and provide you with the extra energy and nutrition you need. Here are some snack ideas for a sample meal plan for pregnancy:

    ☐ Fruits and vegetables: Snacking on fruits and vegetables is an excellent way to get the vitamins and minerals you need. Examples include carrot sticks, apple slices, berries, and sliced cucumbers.

    ☐ Nuts and seeds: Nuts and seeds are a great source of protein, fibre, and other minerals. Examples include almonds, walnuts, chia seeds, and pumpkin seeds.

- [ ] Greek yoghourt: A great source of calcium, which is necessary for strong bones and teeth, is Greek yoghourt. Additionally, it has a lot of protein, which may help you stay satisfied for longer.

- [ ] Hummus and veggies: Hummus is a great source of protein and fibre, and it pairs perfectly with sliced veggies like carrots, celery, and cucumber.

- [ ] Cheese and crackers: Cheese is an excellent source of calcium and protein, and it pairs well with whole-grain crackers.

- [ ] Smoothies: Smoothies are an easy way to pack in nutrients, especially when made with fruits and vegetables like spinach, kale, and berries. You can also add protein powder or Greek yoghurt to make them more filling.

☐ Hard-boiled eggs: Hard-boiled eggs are a convenient and simple snack and a superior source of protein.

It's critical to keep in mind that snacks need to be an addition to your meals, not a substitute. To make sure that you and your baby are getting all the nutrients you need, try to eat a variety of healthful meals throughout the day. Additionally, work with your physician or a qualified dietitian to develop a customised meal plan that takes into account your unique requirements during pregnancy.

3. **Lunch:** Eating a healthy, balanced diet when pregnant is essential for both you and your unborn child's long-term wellbeing. Lunch is a vital meal that can help you meet your nutritional needs. Here

are some ideas for a sample lunch meal plan for pregnancy:

- [ ] Grilled chicken salad: A salad made with grilled chicken breast, mixed greens, tomatoes, cucumbers, and avocado is a great option for a nutritious and filling lunch. Add a drizzle of olive oil and balsamic vinegar for extra flavour.

- [ ] Lentil soup: The high protein and dietary fibre content of lentil soup can help you feel fuller for longer. Iron, which is necessary for producing healthy blood, is also abundant in it.

- [ ] Tuna wrap: A wrap filled with tuna, avocado, lettuce, and tomato provides a healthy dose of protein, healthy fats, and vitamins. You can also add a whole-grain wrap for added fibre.

- [ ] Quinoa bowl: A quinoa bowl topped with roasted vegetables, chickpeas, and feta cheese is a delicious and nutritious lunch option. Quinoa is a complete protein and is high in fibre, making it an ideal choice for pregnancy.

- [ ] Turkey and cheese sandwich: A sandwich made with whole-grain bread, turkey, cheese, lettuce, and tomato is a filling and healthy lunch option. You can also add sliced avocado for extra nutrition.

- [ ] Grilled salmon and veggies: Omega-3 fatty acids are essential for the growth of the developing foetal brain, and grilled salmon is a fantastic source of them. Pair it with roasted or grilled vegetables like broccoli, asparagus, or zucchini for a complete meal.

- ☐ Vegetable stir-fry: It's easy to add flavor and nutrition to a stir-fry by adding veggies like bell peppers, broccoli, carrots, and onions as well as a protein source like tofu or chicken.

Keep hydrated by drinking lots of water throughout the day, and work with your doctor or a qualified dietitian to develop a personalised meal plan that takes into account your particular needs while pregnant.

4. **Dinner:**Dinner is a crucial meal for pregnant women, as it provides the nutrients necessary for foetal growth and development. A well-balanced dinner can also help pregnant women feel full and satisfied, reducing the risk of overeating or

snacking late at night. Here are some ideas for a sample dinner meal plan for pregnancy:

- ☐ Grilled chicken with sweet potato and green beans: Grilled chicken breast is an excellent source of lean protein, which is essential for foetal growth and development. Sweet potatoes are high in fibre and vitamins, while green beans are rich in folate, which is crucial for foetal brain and spinal cord development.

- ☐ Baked salmon with quinoa and roasted vegetables: Omega-3 fatty acids, which are crucial for the growth of the foetus's brain, are abundant in baked salmon. Quinoa is a complete protein and high in fibre, while roasted vegetables like broccoli, cauliflower, and carrots provide a variety of vitamins and minerals.

☐ Lentil stew with whole-grain bread: Iron, which is essential for producing healthy blood, as well as protein and fibre are all found in abundance in lentils. Pair with whole-grain bread for added fibre and nutrition.

☐ Vegetarian chilli with brown rice: A vegetarian chilli made with beans, tomatoes, and peppers is a great source of protein and fibre. Pair it with brown rice, which is high in fibre and B vitamins, for a complete and nutritious meal.

☐ Beef stir-fry with brown rice and vegetables: Beef is a great source of iron, which is essential for foetal blood production. Pair it with brown rice and vegetables like bell peppers, broccoli, and carrots for a complete meal that's high in fibre and vitamins.

- [ ] Black beans, avocado, and baked sweet potato: A baked sweet potato is a great source of fibre and vitamins, while black beans provide protein and fibre. Top with avocado for healthy fats and extra nutrition.

- [ ] Spinach and feta stuffed chicken breast with roasted sweet potato: Stuffed chicken breast filled with spinach and feta cheese is a delicious and nutritious meal. Pair with roasted sweet potatoes for added fibre and vitamins.

Keep hydrated by drinking lots of water throughout the day, and work with your doctor or a qualified dietitian to develop a personalised meal plan that takes into account your particular needs while pregnant. Additionally, it's essential to cook meat and eggs thoroughly to reduce the risk of foodborne illness.

5. **Dessert:**Dessert is often seen as a guilty pleasure, but it can actually be a part of a healthy and well-balanced meal plan for pregnant women. Incorporating nutritious ingredients and choosing low-sugar options can make desserts a healthy and satisfying way to end a meal. Here are some ideas for a sample dessert meal plan for pregnancy:

- [ ] Fresh fruit salad: A bowl of fresh, seasonal fruit is a great option for a healthy dessert. Berries, oranges, and kiwis are all high in vitamin C, which is essential for foetal development.

- [ ] Greek yoghurt with honey and berries: Greek yoghourt is a good source of calcium, which is important for developing a foetus's bones. Drizzle with honey and top with berries for a sweet and nutritious dessert.

- [ ] Baked apples with cinnamon and walnuts: Baked apples are a delicious and healthy dessert option. Sprinkle it with cinnamon and top with chopped walnuts for added nutrition.

- [ ] Chia seed pudding: Chia seeds are a terrific complement to any diet plan since they are packed with fibre and omega-3 fatty acids. Mix chia seeds with almond milk and top with fresh fruit for a delicious and nutritious dessert.

- [ ] Dark chocolate: When consumed in moderation, dark chocolate, which is high in antioxidants, can be a healthy choice. Choose chocolate that is at least 70% cocoa for the most health benefits.

- ☐ Banana ice cream: Frozen bananas blended with a splash of almond milk can create a creamy and healthy ice cream alternative. Top with nuts or dark chocolate for added flavour.

- ☐ Oatmeal cookies with raisins: Oatmeal cookies made with whole-grain oats and raisins are a great source of fibre and iron, which is essential for foetal blood production.

Remember to choose desserts in moderation and be mindful of added sugars. For assistance in developing a customised meal plan that suits your unique needs during pregnancy, speak with your doctor or a qualified dietitian.

REAL FOOD SWAP

To ensure both the mother's and the baby's health and growth throughout pregnancy, it is essential to consume a nutritious and well-balanced diet. However, it can be challenging to make healthy food choices all the time, especially when cravings and hunger strike. One way to make healthier choices is to swap out less nutritious foods for healthier options. Here are some real food swaps for pregnancy:

- [ ] White bread for whole-grain bread: Bread made from whole grains is a fantastic source of fibre and vital nutrients like iron and B vitamins, which are needed during pregnancy. Switching from white bread to whole-grain bread can help you stay full longer and provide lasting energy throughout the day.

- [ ] Processed snacks for whole foods: Processed snacks like chips and crackers are often high in sodium and unhealthy fats. Instead, opt for whole foods like fruits, vegetables, nuts, and seeds, which are packed with vitamins, minerals, and fibre.

- [ ] Sugary drinks for water: Sugary drinks like soda and juice can add extra calories and sugar to your diet without providing any nutritional benefits. Drinking water is essential for staying hydrated and supporting foetal development.

- [ ] Fried foods for grilled or baked foods: Fried foods can be high in unhealthy fats and calories. Instead, opt for grilled or baked options like chicken or fish, which are high in protein and essential nutrients.

- [ ] Cheese for low-fat or reduced-fat options: The growth of a fetus's bones depends on calcium, which is abundant in cheese. However, some types of cheese can be high in fat and calories. Choose low-fat or reduced-fat options to get the benefits of cheese without the extra calories.

- [ ] Ice cream for frozen yoghurt or fruit popsicles: Ice cream is a delicious treat, but it can be high in sugar and calories. Frozen yoghourt or fruit popsicles are a healthier alternative that still satisfies a sweet tooth.
- [ ] Processed meats for lean meats: Processed meats like hot dogs and deli meats can be high in sodium and unhealthy additives. Opt for lean meats like chicken or turkey, which are high in protein and essential nutrients.

Don't forget to work with your doctor or a qualified dietitian to develop a personalized pregnancy food plan that suits your particular requirements. You can make sure that you and your unborn child are getting the nourishment you require for a healthy pregnancy by making easy

substitutions and introducing better options into your diet.

HOW TO SWAP PROCESSED FOOD FOR REAL FOOD DURING PREGNANCY

Processed foods can be convenient and tasty, but they are often high in sugar, unhealthy fats, and additives that can be harmful to both the mother and the baby during pregnancy. Alternatively, genuine foods like fruits, vegetables, whole grains, lean proteins, and healthy fats are brimming with vital nutrients that support foetal development and general health.. Here are some tips on how to swap processed foods for real foods during pregnancy:

☐ Plan ahead: Planning your meals and snacks in advance can help you avoid reaching for processed foods when you're hungry and short on time. Stock up on fresh produce, whole grains, and lean proteins so that you always have a variety of wholesome foods available.

- ☐ Choose whole foods over packaged foods: Instead of packaged meals like chips, crackers, and cookies, choose entire foods like fresh fruits and vegetables, whole grains, and lean meats. Whole foods are often less processed and contain more nutrients and fibre.

- ☐ Read labels: When buying packaged foods, read the ingredient list and nutrition label carefully. Look for foods with fewer ingredients, minimal added sugars, and less sodium.

- ☐ Cook from scratch: Cooking from scratch allows you to control the ingredients and ensure that you are eating real foods. Simple meals like grilled chicken with roasted vegetables or a quinoa salad with fresh herbs and vegetables can be easy and nutritious.

- ☐ Swap out unhealthy fats for healthy fats: Replace unhealthy fats like butter and margarine with healthy fats like olive oil, avocado, and nuts. These fats are high in monounsaturated and polyunsaturated fats, which are important for foetal brain development.

- ☐ Focus on nutrient-dense foods: Nutrient-dense foods like leafy greens, berries, and nuts are packed with vitamins, minerals, and antioxidants. Focus on incorporating these foods into your meals and snacks to ensure that you are getting the essential nutrients you need.

Don't forget to work with your doctor or a qualified dietitian to develop a personalised pregnancy food plan that suits your particular requirements. You can make sure that you and your unborn child are receiving the vital nutrients you require for a healthy pregnancy by substituting natural foods for processed ones.

REAL FOOD SNACK IDEAS

Snacking on real foods is a great way to keep your energy levels up and satisfy hunger between meals during pregnancy. Real foods like fruits, vegetables, nuts, and seeds are packed with essential nutrients that support foetal development and overall health. Here are some real food snack ideas to try:

- Apple slices with almond butter: While almond butter is rich in protein and healthy fats, apples are a fantastic source of fibre and vitamin C.

- Carrots and hummus: Carrots are packed with vitamin A and fibre, while hummus is high in protein and healthy fats.

- Greek yoghurt with berries: Berries are loaded in antioxidants and fibre, while Greek yoghourt is high in calcium and protein.

☐ Trail mix: Mix together nuts, seeds, and dried fruit for a snack that's high in protein, healthy fats, and fibre.

☐ Eggs that have been hard-boiled: Hard-boiled eggs are a fantastic source of protein and key nutrients including choline, which is crucial for the growth of the foetus's brain.

☐ Edamame: Edamame is a great source of protein, fibre, and essential nutrients like folate, which is important for foetal development.

☐ Avocado toast: Top whole-grain bread with mashed avocado for a snack that's high in healthy fats, fibre, and essential nutrients like folate.

☐ Cottage cheese and fruit: Fruit is a fantastic source of fibre and vitamin C, while cottage cheese is a fantastic supply of calcium and protein.

- ☐ Veggie sticks with guacamole: Veggie sticks like carrots, cucumber, and bell peppers are packed with vitamins and fibre, while guacamole is high in healthy fats and essential nutrients like potassium.

- ☐ Homemade energy bars: Make your own energy bars using nuts, seeds, and dried fruit for a snack that's high in protein, healthy fats, and fibre.

Remember to listen to your body's hunger and fullness cues and choose snacks that are nutrient-dense and satisfying. You can make sure that you and your unborn child are receiving the vital nutrients you require for a healthy pregnancy by nibbling on real foods while you are pregnant.

PREGNANCY AND FOOD SAFETY

Food safety is a crucial factor to take into account while pregnant because some meals can harm the developing baby. Foodborne infections can seriously harm both the mother and the unborn child because pregnant women are more prone to them. Here are some tips for ensuring food safety during pregnancy:

- ☐ Wash your hands: Before and after handling food, especially raw meat, poultry, fish, and eggs, it's necessary to wash your hands. This may aid in limiting the spread of dangerous microorganisms.

- ☐ Cook food to the right temperature: By properly cooking food, dangerous microorganisms can be eliminated. Use a food thermometer to check the internal temperature of meat, poultry, fish, and eggs.

☐ Avoid raw or undercooked meat, poultry, fish, and eggs: Raw or undercooked meat, poultry, fish, and eggs can be contaminated with harmful bacteria like salmonella and listeria, which can cause serious illness.

☐ Avoid unpasteurized dairy products: Unsafe bacteria like listeria, which can lead to serious illness, can contaminate unpasteurized dairy products like raw milk and cheese.

☐ Wash fruits and vegetables: Before eating, thoroughly wash fruits and vegetables to get rid of any dirt, bacteria, or pesticides.

☐ Avoid deli meats and hot dogs: Deli meats and hot dogs can be contaminated with listeria, which can cause serious illness. If you do eat deli meats, heat them until they are steaming hot to kill any bacteria.

- [ ] Avoid certain types of fish: Some species, including shark, swordfish, king mackerel, and tilefish, can have high mercury concentrations, which can impair a baby's developing neurological system.

- [ ] Avoid alcohol and caffeine: Alcohol and caffeine should be avoided during pregnancy, as they can have harmful effects on the developing baby.

- [ ] To prevent the growth of hazardous bacteria, store food correctly in the refrigerator at 40°F or lower.

Never forget to talk to your doctor if you have any queries or worries regarding the safety of your diet while pregnant. You can contribute to a safe and healthy pregnancy for you and your unborn child by adhering to these recommendations.

FOOD TO AVOID DURING PREGNANCY

During pregnancy, it is essential to take care of your diet and avoid certain foods that can pose a risk to the health of both the mother and the baby. Here are some foods to avoid during pregnancy:

1. Meat that is either raw or undercooked may include bacteria like Salmonella, E. coli, or Listeria, which can result in life-threatening food-borne infections. These infections can lead to premature delivery, stillbirth, and other complications.

2. Raw or undercooked eggs: Raw or undercooked eggs can also be contaminated with Salmonella bacteria. Foods containing raw eggs, such as homemade Caesar salad dressing, hollandaise sauce, and mayonnaise, should be avoided by expectant mothers.

3. Raw or undercooked seafood: Seafood, such as sushi, sashimi, and oysters, that is raw or undercooked, might harbour dangerous bacteria and parasites. It can lead to foodborne illness and may affect foetal development.

4. Deli meats and hot dogs: Deli meats and hot dogs can be contaminated with Listeria bacteria. Listeria can cause miscarriage, stillbirth, premature delivery, or a serious infection in a newborn baby.

5. Unpasteurized dairy products: Listeria, Salmonella, and E. coli are just a few of the dangerous bacteria that can be found in unpasteurized dairy products including milk, cheese, and yoghurt. Pregnant women should opt for pasteurised dairy products to reduce the risk of infections.

6. Caffeine: Caffeine is a stimulant that can cross the placenta and affect foetal heart rate and breathing.

It is recommended to limit caffeine intake to 200 milligrams a day during pregnancy.

7. Alcohol: Alcohol consumption during pregnancy can result in foetal alcohol syndrome, which can affect the unborn child's physical and mental development. During pregnancy, it is advised to fully avoid alcohol.

In order to lower their chance of contracting a foodborne disease and guarantee a healthy pregnancy, pregnant women should avoid a number of items. It is essential to have a balanced and nutritious diet that includes plenty of fruits, vegetables, whole grains, lean protein, and pasteurised dairy products. If you have any concerns about your diet during pregnancy, talk to your healthcare provider.

CONCLUSION

Eating real, whole foods during pregnancy can provide essential nutrients for both the mother and the growing baby. A nutritious diet that is balanced and diverse and includes a variety of fruits, vegetables, whole grains, lean proteins, and healthy fats can aid in the development of the foetus and lower the chance of difficulties during pregnancy.

Pregnant women should avoid certain foods like raw or undercooked meats, eggs, and seafood, deli meats, and unpasteurized dairy products, which can cause foodborne illnesses and harm the developing baby. It is also recommended to limit caffeine intake and avoid alcohol during pregnancy.

The nutritional needs of a pregnant woman are unique, as her body is working hard to support the growth and development of the foetus. It's important to eat a variety of nutrient-dense foods to ensure the proper intake of essential vitamins, minerals, and macronutrients.

Any special dietary requirements or worries should be brought up with a healthcare professional during pregnancy. Eating a range of real, whole meals can benefit both the mother's and the baby's long-term health and help to promote a good pregnancy.

9 798399 513775